# 21-Day Weight Loss Challenge

## How to Lose 15 Pounds with Low Carb Diet

*FREE BONUS RECIPES INCLUDED!*

The information herein is offered for informational purposes solely, and is universal as so. The presentation of the information is without contract or any type of guarantee assurance.

The trademarks that are used are without any consent, and the publication of the trademark is without permission or backing by the trademark owner. All trademarks and brands within this book are for clarifying purposes only and are the owned by the owners themselves, not affiliated with this document.

# Table of Contents

# Introduction

I want to thank you and congratulate you for buying the book, "*21-Day Weight Loss Challenge: How to Lose 15 Pounds with Low Carb Diet.*"

Weight loss is sometimes a fantasy for most and rarely become a reality for some. Whether your reason is for prevention, cure or aesthetic, weight control is a highly desired goal for most people. While weight loss can truly be a challenge, it does not have to be difficult, especially with the delicious but still low carb recipes under your belt.

This is more than just a 35 recipe book, it is also a guide to give you more than enough information and tips to motivate you towards success in your chosen endeavor of retaking control of your weight. From an overview of the diet, to the secret link between carbs and fats, from ways to prepare and shop for your kitchen and to the actual recipes themselves, every angle is taken accounted for, to help you increase the possibility of your success.

The recipes in this book include:

- 7 beef

- 7 poultry

- 7 seafood

- 7 veggies

- 7 breakfast, snacks and desserts

Plus, the Low Carb Diet, despite being successful at 21 days, does not have to end there. When you have reached your target weight loss at that time, the next step is to sustain your achievement. All your efforts for the past 3 weeks will bear better fruits when you are able to respect your success by maintaining or even improving past the 3 week period.

Thanks again for buying this book, I hope you enjoy it! Don't forget to claim your **FREE BONUS** at the end of this book!

# Chapter 1: Introducing the Low Carb Challenge

## Overview of the Diet

Low carb diets are your best bet to win against the battle for weight control. Healthy eating is one of the strongest foundations to achieve not only weight loss but also total health and wellness. A properly balanced diet, combined with other positive health decision, will result to vast improvements in your health and lifestyle.

When you have a proper diet that takes into account all nutrients you need, from proteins, healthy fats, minerals, vitamins and carbs, then you are one step closer toward achieving your health goals. Diet serves as the fuel to power all your body tissues and organs to maintain its optimum performance. The better your diet is, the better fuel you r body is able to use. Of particular importance is the carb component of your diet.

## Carbs & Weight Control

The low carb diet works because it zeroes in on one of the primary causes of weight gain, the accumulation of fats. The link between carbs and weight gain is found between the transformation of carbs into calories and then into fats. Carbs are meant to power your body throughout the day. When it is consumed, it becomes calories, which is the actual fuel needed by the body to meet your demands. However, when you consume too many calories and your body does not utilize them, for example in a sedentary lifestyle, calories are stored as fats.

This is where the weight control problem becomes apparent. The more carbs you consume and the less activity you do, the more fats are stored and the more weight is gained. When you have low carb consumption, there is less amount of fats to be stored, sometimes you can even consume and expend the exact amount of calories you need for the day.

## Health Benefits & Other Advantages

While the most popular benefit of the low carb diet is the control or reduction of your weight, this benefit is only one of the many advantages of having this kind of diet. Some of the co-morbid illnesses that go with weight gain or obesity include diabetes and hypertension. An added effect of the low carb diet is the reduction of sugar intake, which in turn lowers glucose intake. Low glucose levels are another layer of protection against the occurrence of diabetes and or the decrease in diabetic attacks. With calories controlled, there are less fat deposits, especially in the blood vessels. This allows optimum flow of the blood throughout the rest of the body and prevents constriction arteries or veins, which lowers blood pressure. Other cardiovascular diseases are also either prevented or managed through this diet.

Another set of advantages in the low carb diet belong to the psychological side of health. When you have better control of your health, your physical body feels and looks better. As a result, you may feel more confident or assertive instead of shy or reclusive. You will have a more positive outlook in life.

Take note that extreme weight loss is not part of the objectives of the challenge. Weight control is the best way to determine the best or most ideal weight for your body and unique health background. Never attempt to use the diet to lose too much weight that you end up losing much needed nutrition and energy for your body. Make sure to use the low carb diet responsibly and for your health.

# Chapter 2: Preparing for the Challenge

## Setting Weight Loss Goals

One of the hardest parts of achieving the desired body figure is to start the low carb diet itself. Most people use a goal to motivate them not only to start but also to persist with the diet. However, when a goal is not properly developed or stated, it may lose whatever motivating potential it has. An example of a poorly developed goal is, "I will lose weight." On the other hand, you can make use of a SMART goal. SMART is an acronym that stands for specific, measurable, attainable, relevant and time-bound. To create a better goal, you can say, "By the end of three weeks, I will have lost at least 15 pounds by eating only low carb meals."

Another useful goal is to add the concept of Body Mass Index or BMI. Use the following steps to help you compute the BMI:

To calculate BMI:

1. Weigh yourself using pounds as your measurement
2. Measure your height using inches
3. Multiply the number of inches with itself
4. Divide the result with your weight

5. Multiply the result with 703

For example, if you measure 60 inches and 100 pounds then:

1. 60 x 60 = 3600
2. 100 / 3600 = .03
3. .03 x 703 = 21.09

Refer to the table below to determine your BMI:

18.6 and below = underweight

18.7 to 24.8= ideal weight

24.9 to 29.9 = overweight

30 and above = obesity

Take note of the result of your BMI. If you belong to the opposite extremes of the scale, such as either underweight or obese, it is highly recommended that you consult your doctor on your decision to use the low carb diet.

## Shopping & Restocking the Kitchen

Every little bit of help counts, especially when it is a matter of health. Another effective way to help you succeed in your diet is to prime your kitchen so that you are locked into choosing only the best and healthiest food choices instead of being tempted or accidentally choosing a non-low carb diet food item. This can be best done by resetting your pantry, refrigerator or kitchen into having a low carb stock. On your next trip to the grocery, consider the items below in your shopping list:

For meat: lamb, ham, sirloin steak, roast beef, tenderloin and beef, choose the lean cuts

Poultry: ground turkey, chicken breast and thighs, duck and turkey, remember to remove the skin and fats

Seafood: tilapia, halibut, catfish, tuna, trout, cod, squid and especially salmon

Veggies and fruits: lettuce, arugula, spinach,, potatoes, carrots, avocados, mushrooms, artichokes, radicchio and radish, peppers, celery, cucumber, broccoli, okra, snow peas, brussels sprouts, eggplant and collard greens

Seasonings: parsley, chives, salt, etc.

Others: almond flour, walnuts, goat cheese, cottage cheese, feta and plain yogurt

Refrigerator Staples: eggs, lemon juice, etc.

Take note, some of the healthier versions of this diet will be on the more expensive price range. This is because of the special preparation done to make some of the ingredients above as low carb as possible. Make sure that you prepare not only your list of main ingredients but also your budget.

## Easing Into the Diet

Any abrupt change in your diet increases the risk for failing on your diet. Diet can be overwhelming and confusing but with proper preparation you are a few more steps closer towards your diet goals. Here are some ways to ease into your diet: Gradually remove and replace certain high carb food items in your daily routine. If you are fond of having burgers for snacks or late night ice cream desserts, then you need to reboot your habits. While your 15 pound challenge starts in Day 1, you can have a Week 0 as your preparatory phase. Instead of ice cream, consider yogurt or instead of burgers, consider a fruit snack.

These minor but effective adjustments can prepare you for Day 1 and beyond. Do it step by step. Refrain from the myth of overnight success. There is no such thing as an easy way but every journey begins with a single step. Start with reducing and replacing what you eat.

Drink plenty of water. Water is very important because it eases any hunger pangs and also helps remove the wastes and toxins in your body. It is helpful in your digestion and helps the conversion of food into energy plus it also helps the body to absorb nutrients. Eat lot of vegetables and fruits. This food will help detox and provide nutrients to the body. Make sure to eat the seasonal foods to ensure the freshness and best benefit of it.

# Chapter 3: Your 21-Day Challenge Starts Now!

**Day 1 to 7:** *Start Right, Start Prepared and Start Your Victory*

## Starter Meal Plan A

Breakfast or Snack:
Lemon Square

Lunch :
Meatloaf or Salmon with Cream Sauce

Dinner:
Garlic Chicken or Veggie Meatloaf

## Starter Meal Plan B

Breakfast or Snack:
Walnut Cookies

Lunch:
Pepperoncini and Beef or Egg and Shrimp

Dinner:

Chicken Broccoli or Pizza

Can't wait to start your first challenge and enjoy these delicious low carb meals?

Go to the next page and start cooking away!

## Lemon Square

Start your day with Lemon Squares for breakfast or even snack! Fresh lemon juice is recommended as compared to bottled juice for this recipe. The zest of the lemon definitely adds more flavor to it. These lemon squares are low-carb, sugar-free, and gluten-free.

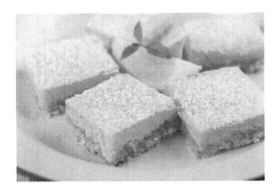

Number of Servings: 18

Ingredients:

- 1/4 cup almond flour
- 1/4 cup powdered xylitol
- 2 tsp sugar substitute
- 4 eggs
- 1/2 cup lemon juice
- 1 cup almond flour

- 1/4 tsp sea salt
- 2 Tbsp powdered xylitol
- 1 Tbsp coconut oil
- 2 Tbsp raw unsalted butter
- 1 Tbsp pure vanilla extract

Instructions:

1) Heat the oven to 350 degrees.
2) Prepare the baking dish.
3) In a large bowl, mix the powdered xylitol, salt and almond flour.
4) In a separate medium sized bowl, put the butter, vanilla extract, coconut oil and mix well.
5) Press the dough into the baking pan evenly.
6) Put inside the oven for 15 minutes or until it turns lightly golden.
7) Prepare another bowl for the toppings.
8) Mix thoroughly the, almond flour, powdered xylitol, stevia, eggs and lemon juice until smoothens.
9) Get the crust inside the oven and spread evenly the toppings over the hot crust.
10) Put again inside the oven for 15 minutes until toppings turn into slightly golden.
11) Cut in squares and serve.

## Meatloaf

This delicious low carb and high protein meatloaf is a comfort food classic! The cheesy, beefy flavor always makes a great meal to prepare for your loved ones and gatherings because it is so quick and easy to make!

Number of Servings: 7

Ingredients:

- 1/2 cup onion, minced
- 1 1/2 tsp salt
- 1 1/2 tsp ground pepper, black
- 2 lbs ground beef
- 3/4 cup bread crumbs
- 2 eggs, beaten
- 3 cups shredded Cheddar cheese

Instructions:

1) Set the heat of the oven to 350 degrees
2) Ready and prepare the beef, bread crumbs, onion, eggs, salt and pepper and mix them in a large bowl.

3) On a large piece of paper, pat out meat mixture into a 14x18 inch rectangle shape.

4) Sprinkle the cheese over the meat, leaving a 3/4 inch border around the edges.

5) Spin and roll up jelly roll fashion to wrap the filling and form a pinwheel loaf.

6) Squeeze or press beef in on both ends to enclose the cheese.

7) Place in a 10x15 inch baking dish.

8) Put inside the oven and bake for 1 hour or until it reaches 160 degrees

9) Serve

## Salmon with Cream Sauce

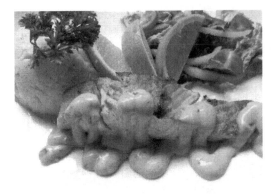

Number of Servings: 4

Ingredients:

- 1 ½ lbs salmon fillets
- ½ cup fat free sour cream
- 1 tbsp olive oil
- 1 garlic clove, minced
- ¼ cup lemon juice
- 2 tbsp capers
- 1 tsp lemon-pepper seasoning

Instructions:

1) Heat the oven to 350 degrees.
2) Grease the baking sheet.

3) Put the oil in the pan and place it over a medium heat.

4) Put the garlic and cook it for 1 minute.

5) Put the heat to low, add in the pan the lemon juice, capers and lemon-pepper.

6) Cook it for 5 minutes.

7) Add the sour cream and cook for another 5 minutes.

8) Place the salmon in the prepared baking sheet.

9) Put inside the oven for 20 minutes.

10) Put the sauce over the salmon.

## Garlic Chicken

Number of Servings: 6

Ingredients:

- 1 tbsp dried parsley
- 6 boneless with skin chicken thighs
- 1/2 cup butter
- 3 tbsp garlic, minced
- 3 tbsp soy sauce

Instructions:

1) Grease the baking pan and heat the oven.
2) Put together the butter, garlic, soy sauce, pepper, and parsley in a bowl.
3) Put the bowl inside the microwave for at least 2 minutes or until the butter is melted.
4) In the baking pan, arrange properly the chicken and coat the butter with mixture.
5) Put the chicken inside the oven for 20 minutes.
6) Lastly sprinkle the parsley before serving.

## Veggie Meatloaf

Number of Servings: 8

Ingredients:

- 2 eggs
- 1/2 tsp garlic powder
- salt and pepper to taste
- 1 (12 oz) packaged vegetarian burger crumbles
- 1 (1 oz) packet beef and onion dry soup mix
- 1/2 cup bread crumbs
- 1 1/2 tsp vegetable oil

Instructions:

1) Heat the oven to 400 degrees.
2) Grease the loaf pan.
3) Beat the egg.
4) In a large bowl, mix together the burger crumbles, bread crumbs, and onion soup.
5) Add the egg, garlic powder, salt and pepper and mix it.
6) Spread the mixture in the prepared loaf pan.
7) Put it inside the microwave oven for about 30 minutes or until it is firmed.

## 8) Walnut Cookies

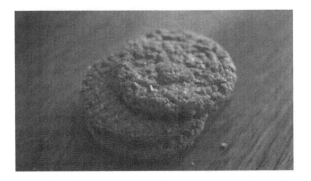

Number of Servings: 1 dozen

Ingredients:

1 (3.9 oz) package instant chocolate pudding mix

1/2 cup chopped walnuts

3/4 cup buttermilk baking mix

1/4 cup vegetable oil

1 egg

Instructions:

1) Heat the oven to 350 degrees.
2) Beat the eggs.
3) In a bowl, put the egg, pudding and vegetable oil.
4) Grease the cookie sheet.
5) Put inside the oven for 10 minutes.
6) Ready to serve the baked cookies.

## Pepperoncini and Beef

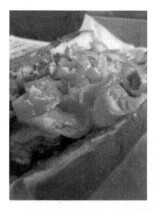

Number of Servings: 7

Ingredients:

- 16 slices provolone cheese
- 4 cloves garlic
- 1 (3 pound) beef chuck roast
- 1 (16 ounce) jar pepperoncini
- 8 hoagie rolls, split lengthwise

Instructions:

1) Slice 4 cloves of garlic.
2) Make small cuts inside the roast and insert garlic slices in the cuts.

3) Put and place the roast in the slow cooker and sprinkle the pepperoncini to the entire content including liquid over the whole meat.

4) Cook on low for 6 to 8 hours. Make sure that the cooker is fully covered.

5) Place the meat in rolls, top with cheese and zap in a microwave for a few seconds when making sandwiches.

6) Put the pepperoncini in the sandwiches.

# Egg and Shrimp

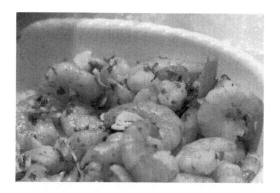

Number of Servings: 2

Ingredients:

- 6 eggs
- 2 t sesame oil
- 1 tbsp soy sauce
- 4 tbsp canola oil
- 1⁄4 cup onion (chopped)
- 2 cups cabbage (shredded)
- 1⁄2 tsp garlic powder
- 1⁄4 tsp salt
- 1⁄8 tsp fresh ground black pepper
- 1 cup bean sprouts (pressed down firmly in cup)
- 1 cup cooked small shrimp (or large dice medium)

Instructions:

1) In a pan, put the 2 tbsp of oil; cook the onions and cabbage over medium high heat.

2) Remove the pan from the heat and drain off excess liquid.

3) Set aside the onions and cabbage

4) Beat the egg in a bowl.

5) Put the sesame oil, soy sauce, spices, onions, sprouts and cabbage mixture inside the bowl and mix it with the egg.

6) Use the pan and heat the 2 tbsp of oil.

7) Put the mixture in the hot pan and sprinkle the shrimp evenly on the top.

8) Cook it for about 3 minutes or until it turns brown.

9) To avoid being overcooked, flip it and wait for another 3 minutes.

10) If the egg turns brown so quickly, use the microwave oven as an alternative to avoid overcooked.

## Chicken Broccoli

Number of Servings: 6

Ingredients:

- 1/2 cup shredded Cheddar cheese
- 1 tbsp butter
- 2 tbsp dried bread crumbs
  1 lbs chopped fresh broccoli
- 1 1/2 cups cubed, cooked chicken meat
- 1 (10.75 ounce) can condensed cream of broccoli soup
- 1/3 cup milk

Instructions:

1) Prepare and heat the oven to 450 degrees.
2) Put the broccoli to a bowl with enough water.
3) Cook it for 5 minutes or until it becomes tender.
4) Place the chicken in a plate and put over the cooked broccoli.
5) In a separate bowl, mix the soup and milk, and pour over the chicken and broccoli.
6) Pour the cheddar cheese.

7) Mix the bread crumbs and butter and sprinkle over the cheese.

8) Put inside the oven for 15 minutes or until it became brown.

## Recipe Name: Pizza

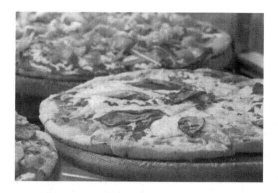

Number of Servings: 24

Ingredients:

- 1/4 cup grated Romano cheese
- 2 tomatoes, sliced
- 1/4 cup grated Parmesan cheese
- 1 readymade pizza crust
- 1/2 cup pesto
- 1 cup ricotta cheese

Instructions:

1) Heat the oven to 450 degrees.
2) In a medium sized bowl, mix the ricotta cheese and parmesan cheese.

3) In the ready to cook pizza crust, spread over the pesto and arrange the tomatoes over the cheese.

4) Put inside the oven for 15 minutes.

## Exercise Challenge

Consider less physically demanding exercises. With the decrease in energy, you will need to conserve your strength until your body adjusts to your new diet. Brisk walking, short distance runs and stationery exercises such as meditation and yoga are your best options for this week of your diet challenge.

Here is an example of a yoga exercise which you can incorporate into your week 1 challenge.

## Half Moon Pose

The benefits of this pose are to tone your buttocks, upper and inner thighs. You will feel the stretch on the sides of your tummy. This will helps in weight loss and burn off those unwanted love handles and strengthen your core at the same time.

**Note: Avoid this pose if you have digestive disorders, a spine injury or high blood pressure.**

Steps:

1) Stand with your feet together.

2) Raise your hands above your head and clasp your palms together, extend the stretch by trying to reach for the ceiling.

3) Exhale, and slowly bend sideways from your hips, keeping your hands together. Remember not to bend forward and keep your elbows straight. You should feel a stretch from your fingertips to your thighs.

4) Inhale and come back to the standing position. Repeat this pose on the other side.

# Day 8 to 14: Keep Going! You're Halfway through the Challenge

## Starter Meal Plan A

Breakfast or Snack:
Brownies

Lunch:
Barbecue Steak or Crab Cakes

Dinner:
Chicken with Spinach or Chili frittata

## Starter Meal Plan B

Breakfast or Snack:
Tarts

Lunch:
Meatballs or Grilled Seafood

Dinner:
Baked Chicken Breast or Veggie Salad

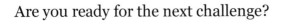

Are you ready for the next challenge?

Go ahead and start planning your week 2 low carb meals!

## Brownies

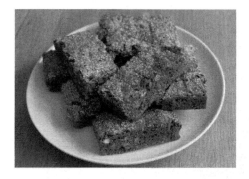

Number of Servings: 25

Ingredients:

- 1 (1.4 oz) package sugar free, chocolate fudge instant pudding
- 1 cup skim milk
- 1/2 cup margarine
- 1/4 cup unsweetened cocoa powder
- 2 eggs
- 1 cup sugar substitute
- 3/4 cup all-purpose flour
- 1/8 tsp salt
- 1/4 cup skim milk
- 1/2 cup walnuts, chopped

Instructions:

1) Heat the oven for 350 degrees.

2) Beat the eggs.

3) Grease the baking pan.

4) Over a medium heat, place the sauce pan and melt the margarine together with the cocoa.

5) Stir it constantly until smooth.

6) Set aside.

7) In a bowl, put the beat eggs, scurrilous sweetener, salt, flour, cocoa and melted margarine.

8) Lastly put the 1/4 cup of milk and the walnuts.

9) Spread into the baking pan the mixture.

10) Bake it inside the oven for 30 minutes.

11) Cool it for 15 minutes.

12) In a separate small bowl, mix for 2 minutes the sugar free chocolate pudding and 1 cup skim milk using electric mixer for frosting.

13) Lastly, spread over the cooled brownies before cutting into squares.

14) Ready to serve the sugar free brownies.

## Barbecue Steak

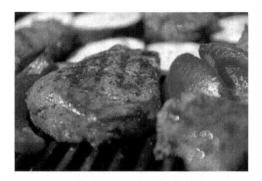

Number of Servings: 6

Ingredients:

- 1/2 tsp ground ginger
- 2 tbsp distilled white vinegar
- 3 tbsp honey
- 1/4 cup soy sauce
- 1/2 tsp garlic powder
- 1/2 cup vegetable oil
- 1 1/2 lbs flank steak

Instructions:

1) Put all together the soy sauce, honey, vinegar, ginger, garlic powder and vegetable oil in a blender.

2) Prepare the steak and put it in a large bowl or ceramic dish, pierce both sides of the steak with a sharp fork, sprinkle the marinade over the steak and make sure that it was fully covered or soaked in the marinade sauce so that it will absorb the flavor.

3) Cover and refrigerate it for 8 hours or overnight.

4) Heat the grill with high heat.

5) Place grate on highest level, and brush lightly with oil.

6) Place steaks on the grill, and discard marinade.

7) Grill steak for 10 minutes, turning once, or to desired doneness.

## Crab Cakes

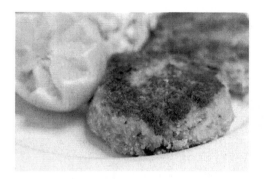

Number of Servings: 2

Ingredients:

- 1 egg
- ¼cup breadcrumbs
- 1 tbsp parsley flakes,
- 2 tbsp mayonnaise
- 2 tsp Worcestershire sauce
- 1 tsp baking powder
- low-carb ketchup
- mayonnaise, for sauce
- 2(6 oz) crab meat, drained
- 1 tsp Old Bay Seasoning

Instructions:

1) Prepare the crabs.

2) Pick over the crab meat for pieces out of their shells.

3) Beat the egg in a bowl and add the parsley, baking powder, Worcestershire sauce, crab meat and mix it.

4) Mold and form 4 patties.

5) Oil the pan and put it over a medium high heat.

6) Cook the crab patties for almost 3 minutes per sides until it turns into golden brown.

7) Serve the crab patties together with the low carb ketchup and mayonnaise.

## Chicken with Spinach

Number of Servings: 4

Ingredients:

2 cloves garlic

4 skinless, boneless chicken breasts

4 slices bacon

1/2 cup mayonnaise

1 (10 ounce) package frozen chopped spinach, thawed and drained

1/2 cup crumbled feta cheese

Instructions:

1) Heat the oven to 375 degrees.
2) Chop the 2 cloves of garlic.
3) Put together the mayonnaise, spinach, feta cheese and garlic in a bowl until mixed properly.
4) Keep aside the bowl.
5) Cut the chicken breast in the middle carefully and put inside the spinach mixture.
6) Use bacon to wrap each piece of chicken breast and secure with a toothpick.
7) Put the chicken breast in a baking dish and cover it.

8) Put it inside the oven for 1 hour or until the chicken turns brown.

## Chili frittata

Number of Servings: 10

Ingredients:

- 1 (7 oz) can diced green chili peppers, drained
- 1 (16 oz) container low-fat cottage cheese
- 1 cup shredded Cheddar cheese
- 1/4 cup butter
- 10 eggs
- 1/2 cup all-purpose flour
- 1 tsp baking powder
- 1 pinch salt

Instructions:

1) Heat the oven to 400 degrees.
2) Beat the eggs.
3) Grease the baking dish.
4) In a bowl, mix the egg, flour, baking powder, salt, chili pepper, cottage cheese, cheddar cheese and butter.
5) Spread into the baking dish.
6) Put inside the oven for 15 minutes.

7) Adjust the heat to 325 degrees and let it be cooked for another 35 minutes.

## Tarts

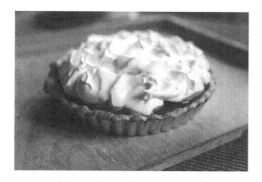

Number of Servings: 24

Ingredients:

- 1/2 cup butter
- 1 cup all-purpose flour
- 3 oz cream cheese

Instructions:

1) Heat the oven to 235 degrees.
2) In a bowl, put the flour, butter and cheese and mix it well.
3) Prepare the dough and mold it into 24 one-inch balls and press it into ungreased muffin cups to make a shell.

4) Put the toppings over the shells and baked it inside the oven for 20 minutes.

## Meatballs

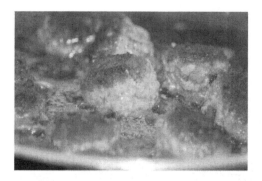

Number of Servings: 4

Ingredients:

- 3 tbsp Worcestershire sauce
- 1 tbsp butter
- 1 tbsp prepared yellow mustard
- 1 tsp red pepper flakes
- 1 tsp Cajun seasoning
- 1 tsp extra virgin olive oil
- 1 tsp lean ground beef
- 3/4 cup crushed seasoned croutons
- 1/4 cup chopped sweet onion
- 1 egg, lightly beaten
- 2 cloves garlic

Instructions:

1) Chop 2 cloves of garlic.
2) Put all together in a large bowl the ground beef, croutons, sweet onion, egg, garlic, Worcestershire sauce, mustard, red pepper flakes, and Cajun seasoning.
3) Form the mixture into meatballs using bare hands.
4) In the frying pan, put the olive oil and melt the butter over a medium heat.
5) Place the meatballs in the frying pan and cook, turning constantly, twenty minutes or to desired doneness.

## Grilled Seafood

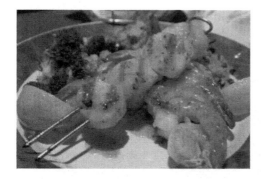

Number of Servings: 6

Ingredients:

- 1 lb scallops
- 1lb shrimp, peeled
- 3cloves garlic, minced
- 2 tsp ground coriander
- 1 tsp ground cumin
- 6 tbsp soy sauce
- ¼cup lime juice
- ¼cup brown sugar
- 2 tbsp olive oil
- 2 tbsp ketchup

Instructions:

1) In a bowl, mix the lime juice, soy sauce, sugar, garlic, oil, ketchup and spices.
2) Marinate the shrimp and scallop for around 1 hour.
3) Make sure to soak the scallop and shrimp properly.
4) Thread the shrimp and scallop onto the skewer after an hour.
5) Cook it over a medium hot grill.
6) Constantly turn it for 3 minutes to avoid being overcooked.
7) Oil it with the marinade while cooking

## Baked Chicken Breast

Number of Servings: 4

Ingredients:

- 4 boneless chicken breast
- 2 tsp dried parsley
- 1/2 cup lemon juice
- 1/2 tsp onion powder
- ground pepper black
- salt

Instructions:

1) Prepare the grill with medium heat. Oil the grate.
2) Soak the chicken in the lemon juice.
3) Sprinkle the pepper, onion powder, salt and dried parsley.
4) On the prepared grill, for 10 to 15 minutes, place the chicken and constantly turn it to avoid being overcooked.

## Veggie Salad

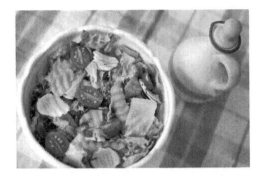

Number of Servings: 8

Ingredients:

- 2 tbsp fat-free mayonnaise
- 1 tbsp fat-free milk
- 1 tbsp sour cream
- 1 garlic clove, minced
- 1 tsp dried oregano
- 1/2 tsp ground cumin
- 1/8 tsp hot pepper sauce
- 1/4 cup chopped green chilies
- 4 cups torn romaine
- 4 cups julienned peeled turnip
- 2 medium tomatoes cut
- 1/2 cup shredded reduced-fat cheddar cheese

Instructions:

1) In a large bowl, put the turnip, tomatoes, cheese, and romaine and mix it.
2) In a separate medium sized bowl, mix the mayonnaise, milk, cream, garlic, oregano, cumin, sauce and chilies.
3) Spread the mixture over the salad.

## Exercise Challenge

Level up on this week's exercises by increasing the intensity of your workout. With renewed energy provided by the adjustment gained by your body on the new diet, you can opt for exercises that can augment your weight loss goals. You can start carrying weights, increasing the speed and distance of your runs and participating in team sports.

## Curl to Press

This strength training targets biceps and shoulders.

1) Hold a dumbbell in each hand and sit on a stability ball or chair with knees bent and feet on the ground.
2) Extend arms at sides, palms facing forward.
3) Curl weights toward shoulders, and then rotate palms away from you as you press dumbbells straight overhead.
4) Reverse the motion to return to starting position.

# Day 15 to 21: Final Stretch to Weight Loss Success! You Did It!

## Starter Meal Plan A

Breakfast or Snack:
Casserole baked Egg

Lunch:
Classic Beef with Salt and Pepper or Seafood Salad

Dinner:
Marinated Broiled Chicken or Mixed Egg, Squash and Cheese

## Starter Meal Plan B

Breakfast or Snack:
Oatmeal

Lunch:
Grilled Beef or Baked Seafood

Dinner:
Chicken Bread or Mixed Tofu

Your last week of challenge is finally here! Since you have come this far, now it is time to hit your weight loss target! Let's do it!

# Casserole Baked Egg, Spinach, Yogurt and Chili Oil

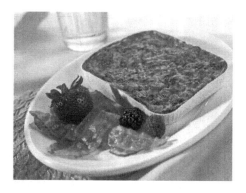

Number of Servings: 2

Ingredients:

- 4 eggs
- 1/4 tsp crushed red pepper flakes and a pinch of paprika
- 1 tsp chopped fresh oregano
- 1 tsp lemon juice
- 2/3 cup plain Greek-style yogurt
- 1 garlic clove
- Kosher salt
- 2 tbsp unsalted butter
- 2 tbsp olive oil
- 3 tbsp leek, chopped

- 2 tbsp scallion, chopped
- 10 cups fresh spinach

Instructions:

1) Heat the oven to 300 degrees.
2) In a small bowl, mix the garlic, salt and yogurt. Set aside.
3) In a large pan, melt 1 tbsp of butter with oil over medium heat.
4) Reduce the heat and make it low, add the scallion and leek.
5) Cook for 10 minutes.
6) Add lemon juice, salt, spinach and turn the heat to high for 5 minutes.
7) Stir it frequently.
8) Transfer the spinach mixture to another pan and leave the excess oil.
9) Divide the spinach mixture equally between the pans.
10) Break the eggs carefully into each pan and make sure not to break the egg yolk.
11) Put inside the oven for 10 minutes.
12) Put the remaining 1 tbsp of butter in the saucepan over medium low heat.

13) Add the salt and pepper for 1 minute then put the oregano.

14) Remove the garlic from the yogurt.

15) Spread the yogurt over the spinach and eggs.

16) Pour the butter.

## Classic Beef with Salt and Pepper

Number of Servings: 7

Ingredients:

- 1 1/2 tbsp all-purpose flour
- 1/2 cup white wine
- 2 cups beef broth, divided
- 3/4 cup crème fraiche
- 1 tbsp fresh chopped chives
- salt and pepper to taste
- 1 tbsp vegetable oil
- 2 lbs beef chuck roast, cut into 1/2-inch thick strips
- salt and pepper to taste
- 1 tbsp butter
- 1/2 medium onion, sliced or diced
- 8 ounces sliced mushrooms
- 2 cloves garlic, minced

Instructions:

1) Pour the salt and pepper to the beef
2) Heat the olive oil in the frying pan over high heat.

3) Put the beef and constantly turn it for 6 to 7 minutes until meat turns to brown and all liquid evaporates.

4) Get the meat and put them in a separate bowl.

5) Put the mushrooms, onions and butter into the frying pan and properly mix it over a medium heat until the vegetables are lightly cooked.

6) Put the garlic and stir for 30 seconds.

7) Mix in flour and cook for 1 to 2 minutes.

8) Add the wine and the cup of stock and scrape the bottom part of the frying pan to remove sticky bits from the pan and avoid being overcooked.

9) Cook thoroughly until it thickens the sauce.

10) Bring back the beef and the remaining cup of stock to the frying pan and mix it.

11) Adjust to low heat and cook it for about an hour until the beef breakable and the sauce is thick.

12) Stir constantly every 20 minutes.

13) Lastly add the crème fraiche and chives. Sprinkle with salt and pepper.

## Seafood Salad

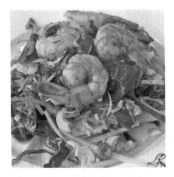

Number of Servings: 2

Ingredients:

- 4 oz cucumber, made into ribbons with a potato peeler leaving seeds
- 1oz shrimp
- 8 oz cucumbers,
- 5ounces radishes
- 1 oz roasted peanuts
- 2 tbsp coriander
- 2 tsp sugar substitute
- 2 oz fish sauce
- 2 oz lime juice
- 1 red chili
- 2 garlic cloves
- 2 tsp ginger root

Instructions:

1) Into a large bowl, put the sugar substitute, fish sauce, lime juice, sliced red chili, garlic, ginger root and mix it well.

2) Slice cucumber into pieces.

3) Put all the remaining ingredients into the large bowl except for the peanut and coriander then mix it.

4) Lastly sprinkle the peanut and chopped coriander on the top.

## Marinated Broiled Chicken

Number of Servings: 2

Ingredients:

- 1 tbsp olive oil
- 1 tbsp red wine vinegar
- 2 skinless, boneless chicken breast
- 1 (1 ounce) package dry Ranch-style dressing mix

Instructions:

1) In a medium sized bowl, mix the vinegar, oil and dressing mix.
2) Put the chicken breast in the bowl, soak properly and cover it.
3) Refrigerate it for almost 8 hours or overnight
4) Get the chicken and put inside the microwave for about 15 to 20 minutes or until it turns brown.

## Mixed Egg, Squash and Cheese

Number of Servings: 8

Ingredients:

- 2 tbsp white sugar
- 2 tbsp all-purpose flour
- 1/4 tbsp salt
- 1/4 tsp ground black pepper
- 6 tbsp butter, melted
- 2 tbsp vegetable oil
- 3 summer squash, sliced
- 1 small onion, diced
- 4 eggs, beaten
- 2 tbsp milk
- 3 cups shredded Cheddar cheese

Instructions:

1) Heat the oven to 375 degrees.
2) Put the oil in a large pan and place it over a medium heat.
3) Put the squash and onion for 10 minutes and stir constantly.

4) In a medium sized bowl, mix the milk, sugar, cheddar cheese, egg, flour, salt and black pepper.

5) Add the squash and melted butter with the 2 remaining cups of cheddar cheese.

6) Put inside the oven for 40 minutes.

## Oatmeal

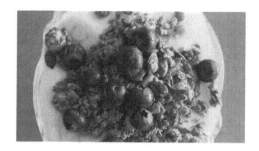

Number of Servings: 4

Ingredients:

- ½ cup and 2 tbsp chia seeds
- ½ cup and 2 tbsp golden flax meal
- ½ cup and 2 tbsp finely shredded unsweetened coconut
- 1 Tbsp and ¾ tsp ground cinnamon
- ½ cup hot water
- 2 Tbsp unsweetened coconut milk
- Sweetener/honey

Instructions:

1) In a bowl, put the chia seed, unsweetened coconut, flax meal, cinnamon and mix it.

2) In a separate bowl, scoop out 1/4 cup of oatmeal.

3) Put 1/2 cup of water over the oatmeal mixture and let it be for 5 minutes.

4) Add the sweetener and 2 tbsp of cream into the bowl and mix it.

5) Lastly, pour the toasted coconut and berries.

## Grilled Beef

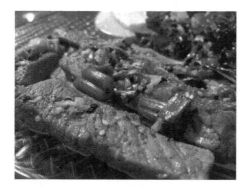

Number of Servings: 7

Ingredients:

- 2 cloves garlic
- ground black pepper to taste
- 4 lbs beef tri tip, cut into 1/2 inch slices
- 1/4 cup soy sauce
- 1/4 cup olive oil
- 2 tbsp water

Instructions:

1) Heat the oven.
2) Peeled and chopped 2 cloves garlic.

3) Mix the soy sauce, olive oil, water, garlic and pepper in a large bowl.

4) Put the beef in the marinade sauce.

5) Soak the beef and cover the bowl.

6) Put in the refrigerator the marinated beef.

7) For 3 to 5 minutes per side, grill the beef slices.

## Baked Seafood

Number of Servings: 8

Ingredients:

- 1lb sea scallops
- 1lb shrimp, shelled and cleaned
- 1/4cup chives
- 1/4cup flour
- 1cup light cream
- 1 1/2cups cracker crumbs
- 3 tbsp butter
- 2cups water, lightly salted
- 1/2cup white wine
- 1sprig fresh dill
- 1/4cup butter
- 4 oz fresh mushrooms

Instructions:

1) Boil the wine, dill and water.
2) Put the scallop and simmer it for 2 minutes.
3) Put the shrimp and simmer it for 3 minutes.
4) Put the seafood in a plate and reserve the liquid.

5) Put the butter in a pan and heat it.

6) Heat the mushroom with chive or green onions into the hot pan.

7) Add the flour and continue cooking up to 1 minute.

8) Add the cream and 1 cup of fish stock.

9) Slowly cook it until thickens.

10) Add the salt and pepper.

11) Pour the sauce over the seafood.

12) Get a separate small bowl and mix the melted butter and cracker crumbs.

13) Sprinkle the mixed butter and cracker crumbs over the seafood.

14) Put inside the oven for 15 minutes or until it turns light brown.

## Chicken Bread

Number of Servings: 6

Ingredients:

- 3 tbsp butter
- 1/2 cup finely crushed herb-seasoned stuffing mix
- 1 tbsp Italian-style seasoning
- 6 boneless chicken breasts
- 3 tbsp grated Parmesan cheese
- 1 tbsp dried parsley
- 1 tsp curry powder

Instructions:

1) Heat the oven to 350 degrees.
2) Mix together in a bowl the cheese, parsley, stuffing mix, curry powder and seasonings.
3) In a separate bowl, put the butter and melt it inside theo oven.
4) Put the chicken breast in the stuffing mixture; make sure it will be fully coated.

5) Place the chicken in the second bowl with melted butter and pour all the left over stuffing mixture over the chicken.

6) Put inside the oven the chicken pieces for 30 minutes to be cooked.

## Mixed Tofu

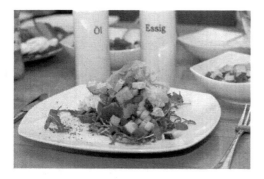

Number of Servings: 4

Ingredients:

- ground turmeric to taste
- salt and pepper to taste
- 1/2 cup shredded Cheddar cheese
- 1 tablespoon olive oil
- 1 bunch green onions, chopped
- 1 (14.5 oz) can peeled and diced tomatoes with juice
- 1 (12 oz) package firm silken tofu, drained and mashed

Instructions:

1) Put the olive oil in a pan and place it over a medium heat.

2) Put the onions for 3 minutes.

3) Add tomatoes with juice and mashed tofu.

4) Sprinkle pepper, salt and turmeric.

5) Reduce the heat and pour cheddar cheese and serve.

## Exercise Challenge

By this time, your weight loss will have reached its optimum and steady level. You can now make full use of your energy gained from your low carb diet. Test your limits by undergoing topnotch exercises, such as surpassing your Week 2 averages. Consider sports that pit you against yourself, few of the best examples are swimming and long distance biking.

Here are some quick tips for long distance biking.

1) Wear the proper clothing.

2) Pack an emergency kit.

3) Pack high energy foods and water.

4) Work your way up to longer distances. Start with shorter trips close to home.

5) Plan your route.

6) Warm up and stretch for ten minutes before you begin.

7) Stick to a comfortable pace. Cycle at a pace which suits you and try to keep this pace as best you can.

8) Adjust your gears.

9) Stop every 10–20 miles (16–32 km) depending on your abilities. Consume some water and food. Check your bike for any problems. Take breaks along the way until you reach your destination.

10) Rehydrate and cool down after you finish.

# Chapter 4: Day 22 & Beyond

## What's next?

One you have reached your target weight after your 21 day challenge, what is next? Most people will assume that those who are successful in the diet will revert to old ways. However, the opposite is actually true. Those who are successful with the diet will enjoy the results so much that they will use it as motivation to sustain the diet. You should too!

Once your body reaches its ideal weight, you need to respect the achievement. Make it a point to discipline yourself and sustain the results of your efforts by making a plan for Week 4 and beyond.

## Tweak your Meals, Plan your Activities

Make your recipes more interesting by changing the main ingredients for a completely different meal. Add in your plan, physically engaging activities such as exercises, walks in the park, and training in the gym or participating in a sport. These activities will burn whatever excess calorie that you have preventing the accumulation of fat deposits, which will contribute greatly to your weight control and total wellness.

# Chapter 5: Managing Your Expectations

## Physical Changes

During the first week of the challenge, especially the first to third days, you can expect no major changes in your body or energy. However in the later part, the most noticeable change is the decrease in energy. You will feel that you get tired easily. This is because of the lowered calorie amount in your body. Do not worry; this is a normal occurrence and temporary. The next week of the challenge, expect to find your body adjusted to your new diet. Due to the optimum working condition of your cells and organs, you will actually feel more energized than ever.

## Psychological Changes

Aside from the temporary decrease in energy, you will also encounter hunger pangs or cravings for carb. This is also normal because your body has become so used to the consumption of carbs that it will trigger your brain to search for the food items. This is very difficult, especially during the first two weeks of the challenge. As much as you can, try to resist the temptation. You can recruit the help of your friends to keep you on track on your diet. You can also substitute your usual carb routines into a healthier alternative. By Week 3, expect your body and appetite to normalize, seeking only the low carb diet that you have been preparing.

## Weight Changes

Of course, weight loss will not happen overnight. Expect the first 3 to 5 pounds to be lost during the latter part of Week 1. Another 4 to 5 pounds will be tapered off during Week 2 and your target 15 pounds or more will be the total loss after the 3 week challenge. Remember, depending on your health background, this weight loss numbers may be different to you.

Keep monitoring your weight changes, one to twice a week. Losing no weight is bad but losing too much is also bad, perhaps even worse. Try to weight yourself once or twice a week to monitor the progress of your weight loss. For diets such as the Low Carb diet, it is best to consult your doctor. Give him the notice that you plan to use this diet and ask for his professional opinion.

# Bonus Recipes

## Pancakes

Number of Servings: 12

Ingredients:

- 2 eggs
- 3 tbsp fat coconut milk
- ½ mashed ripe banana
- ½ tsp apple cider vinegar
- ½ tsp vanilla extract
- 1½ tbsp of coconut flour
- ½ tsp cinnamon
- ¼ tsp baking soda
- salt
- ghee or coconut oil

Instructions:

1) Beat the eggs.
2) In a bowl, mix well the mashed banana, coconut milk, egg, apple cider vinegar and vanilla.

3) In a separate bowl, except for the ghee, mix the remaining ingredients.

4) Mix the 2 mixtures.

5) Grease the pan and add 1 tbsp of butter over a medium heat.

6) Put the mixture into the pan and form a medium sized circle.

7) Bake it for 1 to 2 minutes until bubbles formed in the surface.

8) For another 30 seconds, bake the other side.

9) Pour the butter and ready to serve.

## Pizza

Number of Servings: 8

Ingredients:

- 6 ounces deli sliced corned beef, cut into strips
- 1 (1 lbs) loaf frozen whole wheat bread dough, thawed
- 1/2 cup Thousand Island dressing
- 2 cups shredded Swiss cheese
- 1 cup sauerkraut - rinsed and drained
- 1/2 teaspoon caraway seed
- 1/4 cup chopped dill pickles

Instructions:

1) Heat the oven to 375 degrees.
2) Make sure to grease the pizza pan to avoid sticking with the dough.
3) Form the dough and make a circle with a 14 inches size.
4) Transfer the formed circle dough in the pizza pan.
5) Put inside the oven and bake for 20 to 25 minutes.
6) Pour and spread the dressing salad over the hot crust.

7) Sprinkle 1 cup Swiss cheese, corned beef and the remaining salad.

8) Pour the sauerkraut and remaining Swiss cheese together with the caraway seed.

9) Arrange properly the toppings and seasonings.

10) For another 10 minutes, bake again until cheese melts and toppings are heated.

11) Lastly before slicing, sprinkle the pickles.

## Buttered Chicken

Number of Servings: 4

Ingredients:

- 3 minced cloves garlic
- 4 boneless chicken breasts
- 1/2 cup butter,
- 1 tsp dried parsley
- 1/4 tsp dried rosemary
- 1/4 tsp dried thyme

Instructions:
1) Heat the oven to 350 degrees
2) Put the chicken breast in a pan.
3) In a medium sized bowl, put the garlic, parsley, rosemary, butter thyme and mix it.
4) Spread the mixture on each of the chicken breast.
5) Put inside the oven for about 15 minutes or until it turns brown.

## Fried Seafood

Number of Servings: 4

Ingredients:

- 1 garlic clove
- ½ tbsp lime juice
- salt and pepper
- 3 tbsp olive oil
- 8 oz squids cut to rings
- 4 oz scallops
- 4 oz shrimp, peeled
- 1 tsp chili pepper flakes
- 1/4 tsp cayenne pepper
- 1 tsp Italian seasoning

Instructions:

1) In a bowl, put the chopped garlic, lime juice, salt and pepper, squid rings, scallops, peeled shrimp, chili pepper flakes, cayenne pepper, Italian seasoning and mix it.
2) Put the oil in a large pan and place it over a medium high heat.
3) Fry the seafood mixture for 5 minutes.

## Toasted Eggplant Salad with Almonds and Cheese

Number of Servings: 4

Ingredients:

- 4 garlic cloves
- 2 tbsp of lemon juice
- 1 tbsp soy sauce
- 1 cup flat parsley leaves
- 1/2 cup smoked almonds
- 2 oz goat cheese
- 1/4 cup scallions
- 2 eggplants
- Salt
- 1/3 cup olive oil
- 2 tbsp cider vinegar
- 1 tbsp honey
- 1 tsp smoked paprika
- 1/2 tsp cumin

Instructions:

1) Heat the oven to 400 degrees.
2) Chop the 4 garlic cloves.

3) Chop the parsley leaves.

4) Chop the almonds.

5) Chop the scallions.

6) In a bowl, put the eggplant sliced into 1 inch.

7) Sprinkle the salt and set it aside and make the marinade.

8) In a separate bowl, mix together the vinegar, olive oil, cumin and paprika.

9) Add the garlic into the marinade.

10) Place the eggplant in a baking pan and cook in inside the microwave oven for 15 minutes.

11) Soak the eggplant into the marinade mixture and add the lemon juice, parsley leaves, almonds, scallions and cheese.

# Conclusion

Thank you again for buying this book!

I hope that through this book, you have learned how to maximize the advantages of the low carb diet, especially through the use of the many recipes that are perfect for your weight loss objectives. Remember to make SMART objectives and monitor your progress. Also, it is important that you make a routine of checking your weight as you go through your challenge.

When you have perfected your low carb cooking skills, it is now time to tweak and make recipes of your own. The only limit to your recipes is your creativity. If you keep in mind the carb contents of your ingredients, then you are more than ready to create recipes that are low carb and at the same time suit your preferences.

As soon as you finish reading this book, the next step is to start the preparatory week of your challenge. Prime your pantry and kitchen for success. Ease out of your daily carb loading routine and slowly but surely replace bad with good eating habits. Once you are fully prepared, you are more than ready to start with the 21 day challenge.

With low carb diets and recipes, achieving your weight target is more than possible; it will turn to reality in as short as 21 days.

## Final Thoughts...

Finally, if you received value from this book, please take the time to share your thoughts and post a review on Amazon. It'd be greatly appreciated!

Thank you and good luck!

# Check Out My Other Books

Below you'll find some of my best-selling books that are popular on Amazon and Kindle as well. Simply visit my Author page or search for these titles on the Amazon website to find them.

Get access to ALL my books here,
**http://bit.ly/sarahdawson**

## Diabetes Diet: Ultimate Diabetic Cookbook - Top Most Delicious Recipes to Help You Get Started on Diabetes Diet

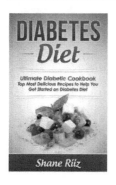

It's a hard blow to find out you have diabetes or even pre-diabetes. When you hear your doctor explain the challenges you're facing, you know your life will never be the same again. One of the changes you probably need to make is the foods you choose to eat. Adopting a diabetic diet is the surest way to get your diabetes under control and start feeling better again.

So, what is a diabetes diet? The main feature of this type of diet is that you need to eat fewer carbohydrates. In fact, many diabetics are encouraged to follow a plan called "carb counting." When you count carbs, you simply add up the carbohydrate servings each time you eat and don't exceed a certain number of servings based on your caloric needs.

While carb counting is effective in reducing the amount of sugar in your bloodstream, many people find that it isn't enough. About 8 to 12 hours after you've eaten a meal loaded with excessive amounts of unhealthy fats, your blood sugar tends to rise significantly. So, for most people, it's also important to limit fat servings.

## The Migraine Cure: Causes of Migraine and the Ultimate Solutions to Relief Your Migraine for Life

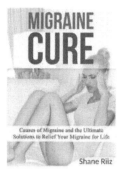

What is a migraine? Everyone, at least once in their life, has confronted with a very bad headache that often tended to reappear. It is a public health issue of strong impact on both the sufferer and society.

To clear your doubt, migraine is defined as a chronic neurological disorder characterized by repetitive mild to intense headaches, frequently in association with some neurological symptoms. It may appear only once every few years or several times a week. It can last between a couple of hours and three days. The pain generally begins in the first part of the day, on one half of the head. (Actually, the word "migraine" is borrowed from a Greek word that means "half-head.") Rarely, the entire head is filled up with pain.

Associated symptoms might include vomiting, nausea, photophobia, sonophobia, or osmophobia. The pain usually gets worse by physical activity. More than one-third of people with migraine headaches sense an aura: a temporary visual, language, sensory or motor interference which indicates that the headache will soon appear. Sometimes an aura can come with brief or no headache succeeding it.

Migraines are considered to be caused by a combination of environmental and inheritable factors. Modifying hormone levels might play a role too, as migraines have more slightly effect on boys than girls before pubescence, but about three times more on women than men. The threat of migraines usually diminishes during pregnancy. The precise mechanisms of migraine are unknown. It is, although, believed to be a neurovascular condition. The main theory is associated with the intensification regarding excitability of the cerebral cortex and irregular control of pain neurons within the trigeminal nucleus belonging to brainstem.

## Paleo Diet: Ultimate Paleo Cookbook for Effective Weight Loss and Healthy Living with Delicious Paleo Recipes

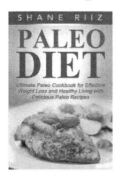

The Paleo diet is one the few diets that is slowly but surely gaining worldwide acceptance. Its success can be credited to its unique take on the proper diet that is best for consumption. The basic foundation of the diet is found on the Paleolithic era or most commonly known as the Stone Age. The idea behind the diet is that our human ancestors, the cavemen, are one of the most physically fit humans to have every walked the face of the earth. The secret behind the cavemen's ability is their source of nutrients and energy.

During those ancient times, the caveman diet consisted primarily of all natural foods. The food was neither processed nor refined. The contents of the diet were also low on sugar and dairy. The major food groups, which were also the only ones available at that time, were those that were naturally growing in the environment of the caveman. These were simple meats, vegetables, fruits, nuts and seeds.

Fast forward to our modern time, our food options are now littered with some of the unhealthiest food in history. High cholesterol fast foods, high sugar content sweets, high sodium preserved foods and other refined and processed foods make up the daily intake of people today. The problem is despite these changes in our food options; our genetic make-up remains the same as with our cavemen ancestors. These means our dietary needs remain the same.

Another problem with the food options today is that even if you buy meats, vegetables, or fruits in the hope that they will be similar to the caveman's own food options, it will rarely be the case. For example, while meat before was grass-fed, today artificial feeds and chemicals are fed or injected to cows, pigs, chicken, fish and other sources of food. While vegetables grew using the natural nutrients of the soil and earth, today there are grown using fertilizers and protected using pesticides.

The solution that the Paleo diet offers is simple, to achieve the same health, endurance and overall well-being of the cavemen, we need to choose only food items that bear the closest resemblance to their diet. This means grass-fed meats, organic vegetables and fruits and other healthier options. It is fortunate that these specialty products are becoming more and more available to the average consumer.

Although the term Paleo diet can be credited to Walter Voegtin, a doctor and gastroenterologist in 1975, it was Joseph Knowles in 1913, who first presented the idea of the benefits of an all natural diet. By immersing himself in the hunger and gatherer lifestyle for 2 whole months, he emerged with a better health and a stronger body.

# Claim Your FREE Bonus!

As a token of appreciation for buying my book, I would like to give away a **FREE BONUS** report, *"10 Quick Weight Loss Tips and Tricks Revealed!"* just for you! May you gain more valuable insights in achieving your weight loss goals!

To claim your FREE bonus, simply go to the URL below:
**http://bit.ly/weightloss-freebonus**

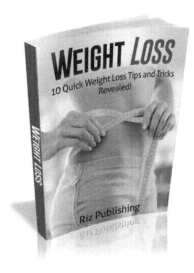

Plus, by signing up to our subscription, you will also receive **FREE KINDLE BOOKS**, recipes, tips and tools to help you attained the weight you desire.

See you on the inside!

Made in the USA
Middletown, DE
29 November 2015